Rapid Weight Loss Hypnosis Tips And Tricks

A Self-Help Guide To Understanding How Close Your Eyes, Get The Body You Want, Pull Your Brain Back To Lose Weight

Self Help for Women Academy

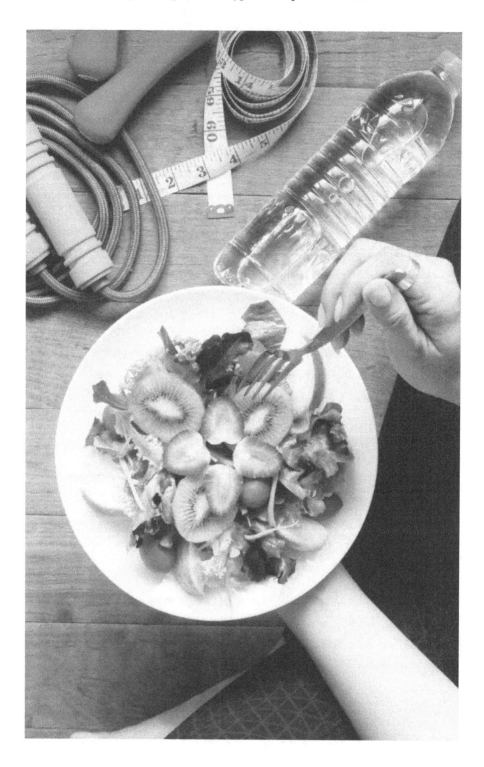

Table of Contents

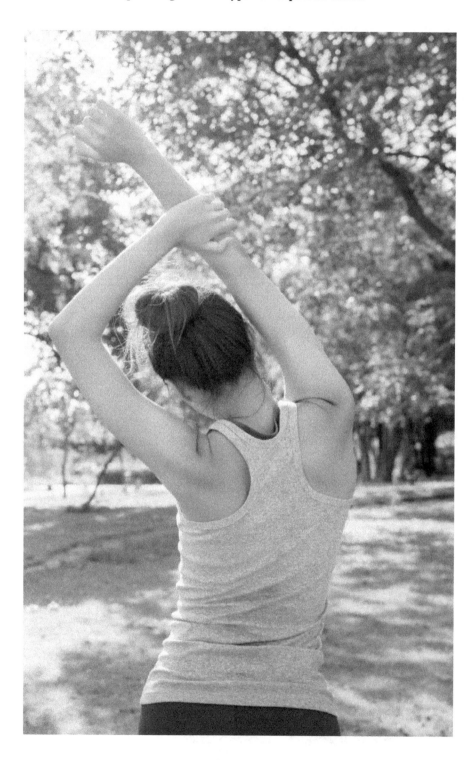

Introduction

Weight loss, in the medical field, refers to a reduction in the total mass of the body; this is caused by the reduction of fluids, fat mass (body fat and fatty tissue), and lean mass (i.e., mineral deposits in the bone, muscle, tendons and other connective tissues).

Weight loss can occur either unintentionally, due to a disease, or for conscious effort and to improve the state of real (or perceived) overweight/obesity.

The so-called "unexplained weight loss," that is, not caused by the reduction in caloric intake than energy expenditure (voluntary or not), is called cachexia and can be a serious medical symptom.

Intentional weight loss is commonly identified as weight loss but, in compliance with what is mentioned in the introduction, represents a different cachexia process.

How to estimate weight loss in the medical field? Unintentional weight loss can result from actual weight loss (fat mass depletion), or loss of bodily fluids, muscular atrophy, or even a combination of these elements. Involuntary weight loss is considered a medical problem when it occurs: at least 10% of the total mass in six months, or at least 5% in the last month.

Another medical criterion used to estimate the total weight (in normal adult subjects, not in children, let alone in athletes) is body mass index (BMI). This provides for the patient's classification to the whole of one of the following categories (representatives of the ranges): underweight, normal weight, and overweight. It follows that, within the same category, a rather important variation can take place (e.g., 10kg). On the other hand, in some older adults, similar or even lower norm weight fluctuations can be much more worrying than interpreted by BMI.

What are the characteristics of inadvertent weight loss? Involuntary weight loss can occur due to an insufficiently nutritious diet as a result of malnutrition. They can also cause unintentional weight loss: pathological processes, changes in metabolism, hormonal changes, drugs or other treatments, pathological evolutions, and reduced appetite.

Intestinal malabsorption can lead to involuntary weight loss caused by fistulas, diarrhea, drug-nutrient interactions, enzyme absence or insufficiency, and mucous membrane atrophy. As anticipated, involuntary, progressive, and wear-and-tear weight loss is sometimes referred to as cachexia. This also differs from slimming for the presence of a systemic inflammatory response and is often related to unfavorable diagnostic results.

In the advanced stages of progressive disease, metabolism can change, leading to weight loss, also utilizing a balanced diet without inducing an increase in the sense of hunger. This condition takes the name of cachexia anorexia syndrome (ACS), often impossible to treat even through supplementation.

Symptoms of involuntary weight loss for ACS include severe muscle depletion, inappetence, and a sense of early satiety, nausea, anemia, weakness, and fatigue.

Involuntary weight loss is a diagnostic criterion for cancer, type 1 diabetes mellitus, thyroid discomfort, etc. What effects can severe involuntary weight loss have?

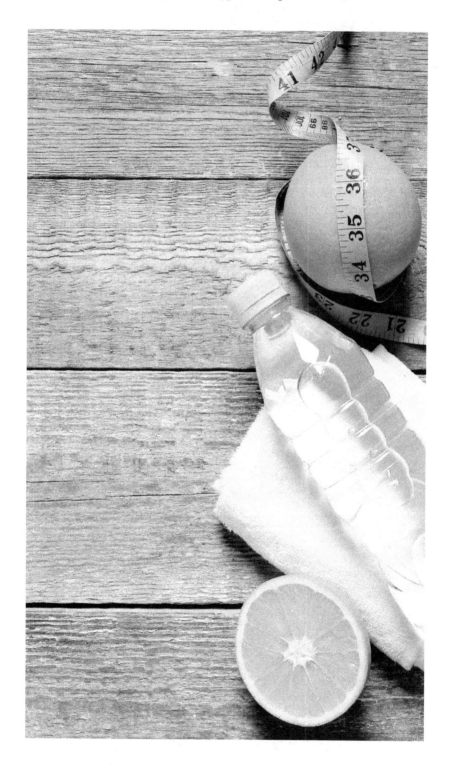

Chapter 1.

Mini Habits for Weight Loss

Good Habits to Lose Weight Without Diet

Here you have small strategies to cheat laziness and not give in to gluttony without stress and too much abstention.

The costume test, as we now know, is being prepared in January.

To show up on time and fit at the summer dress appointment, it takes time and method so that you can gradually weigh weight and not have to get on your toes on the eve of departure for the holidays.

By the way, slowly losing weight is less stressful and tiring for the body, and helps avoid the yoyo effect, according to which at the end of the diet all the lost kilos are taken, moreover with interest.

Here are some good habits that save the line and be adopted permanently until our lifestyle is transformed more healthily.

- **Eating less and moving more:** From this equation, unfortunately, there is no escaping: if we have to lose weight, we need to consume more calories than we introduce with nutrition. A little diet and healthy physical activity must go hand in hand: training, however intense it may be, can make us dispose of superfluous pounds if we do not associate it with a healthy and light diet. Diet alone, to be effective, must be quite restrictive: a fair balance is an ideal solution.

- **Questions of motivation:** If we have to dispose of a certain number of kilos, it is better not to hurry. Let's set ourselves the goal of losing three kilos in a month (it's almost a pound a week, a result that's nonetheless respectfully). If we move with the method and with some care, we will find those food waivers will not be a burden and will not require superhuman willpower. The important thing is to decide that this is our objective and that we will undoubtedly achieve it. We're already getting there. Let's not get haunted by the calorie count and weigh every three to four days, not more.

- **Look for help:** If we do not know how to do it and doubt that our eating habits are not correct, let us inform ourselves. We can ask for the help of a nutritionist or read a good book on the subject. However, if we decide to do it ourselves, let us avoid the regimes that promise to lose many kilos in a short time: these are unbalanced diets that will then make us regain all the weight kilos in a very short time as soon as we start eating normally again.

- **Eat a little bit of everything:** You don't need to eliminate food from our diet. If we do not have bad habits to correct, just decrease the number of portions. The only foods to be banned are those that provide "empty calories," that is, in the absence of beneficial nutrients for the body. This category includes spirits, carbonated and sweetened drinks (including fruit juices), and sweets. If we really can't help it, we can indulge in a couple of squares of dark chocolate once a week. Fruit should be consumed in moderation, better if it breaks hunger in the middle of the morning or at a snack, choosing the less sugary varieties.

- **Tactical dispensation:** Before we go on a diet, let's make what can tempt us to disappear from the pantry and refrigerator. We make a habit of making a list of what the supermarket needs, and when we shop, let's stick to our list without visiting the lanes that can tease the gluttony too much.

- **Let's imagine ourselves lean:** Even if our diet is still in full swing, we will feel more "deflated" and lighter after a few days. We focus on that feeling and learn to look at ourselves in that lean, toned, and active form. When we start to feel the clothes widening, we take the opportunity to gratify ourselves with a new garment, which showcases our line. It will also be the incentive to maintain the good results achieved.

- **Don't skip meals:** It's not a good strategy: it just serves to get hungry to the next meal, where we'll eat a lot more. If we are besieged by the short time, let's organize to prepare a healthy meal in advance and, for example, for lunch at the office, take it with us from home, or we leave dinner ready from the night before if we know we do not have time to cook on the way home. Breakfast is also important: better not to skip it, but at the same time let's be careful not to overeat: a cup of coffee or tea with a slice of toasted wholemeal bread with a little jam without sugar, or a portion of unsweetened whole grains, or a squeeze of fruit or low-fat yogurt are enough to have the right energy without weighing us down.

- **Full plate:** A trick for not overdoing it with portions is to use small plates: a middle portion will be enough to "fill" it and satisfy the view. We create beautiful and colorful dishes, remembering that vegetables, raw or cooked, are our best ally. However, this does not apply to potatoes, which contain starch and are, therefore, assimilated into carbohydrates.

- **What movement:** If doing sports amuses us, we remember not all disciplines are equally effective for burning calories. Cardio and high-intensity fitness are the most useful, but if they are not for us, remember that a fast-paced walk is a great aerobic workout (as long as you keep a sufficient speed, without interruption, at least 40 minutes). Alternatively, we can swim, do aqua-gym, or dance and Zumba. To burn the bearings, you need at least three workouts a week, but we must remember to walk for at least thirty minutes on rest days.

Early Morning Tricks to Lose Weight Quickly

If the situation is familiar to you, then I fully understand why you clean up so often!

That feeling when you are already aware in the early morning that you have made a huge mistake and understand that you have thrown another day of your journey to the nettles towards a spectacular transformation. Turn around, lose motivation, and don't realize the mistakes you've made.

Then you feel guilty, without energy, disappointed. But you continue to dream of a completely different beginning of the day: a morning during which you will know that you are on the right track and feel that your transformation is practically guaranteed. Believe me, and you're not the only one who thinks so. For many, an unachievable dream; for you, a winning routine. But let us now move on to the good news: together, we can make these dreams a reality! And all this by bringing only four very simple habits to your daily routine. Read on to find out which ones. Try to start as early as tomorrow morning!

Well, And if you want to change, starting a day in a new way is no different at all. It is true; however, everything changes if you follow some already tried and tested advice.

And since I want you to live every day as a great opportunity to achieve your fantastic transformation, let me reveal to you the four tricks that will change your morning routine forever and thanks to which you will love the first hours of the day in madness. Don't you believe me? Then let yourself be convinced in the next lines. I'm starting to reveal a particular thing. The perennial question, always the same dilemma. Do you have to have breakfast to burn fat residues and shape a healthy body?

Frankly, the answer is easy. Not! You can also get the desired results by skipping the first meal of the day. There is no doubt about that, and who says otherwise mind. But wait! It's probably also possible to climb Everest in sandals, don't you think?

However, you know that it will be easier to reach the summit wearing the right equipment: in addition to allowing you to reach the summit, the right footwear will allow you to do it more comfortably and simply. And the same goes for a spectacular transformation. Since it is essential to sculpt your body healthily, make you enjoy at all times of your transformation, and let you have enough energy to face all the challenges without problems, I propose another question.

The question that radically changes opinion on lightning transformation here. Is it true that the optimal breakfast is crucial to quickly burn excess fat, get better results, and ensure success? At this point, my answer is completely different. According to various studies, breakfast is one of the most important meals for a lightning transformation. Wait, though! All this only applies if you make a smart choice. But before I reveal the best options, I have another very important piece of information in store for you!

Let's think a moment when most of us do as soon as we hear the alarm ringing. Either we simply skip breakfast because we don't have time, we rush, we're too tired in the morning, or we choose to enjoy a meal rich in simple sugars, such as processed corn or chocolate flakes, croissants, toast, pastries, and other "fast foods."

And what's going on? Both choices harm our hormonal balance. That is why people have to fight hunger attacks, lack of energy, exhaustion, and poor concentration. If you don't believe me, then look at your work colleagues or classmates. I'm sure you'll notice the difficulties listed right away. But it is possible that you too suffer from the same symptoms!

So remember the golden rule: If your goal is to transform the body and enjoy great health quickly, you need to have breakfast within 20 minutes of the moment you wake up. In this way, you introduce quality proteins, healthy fats, and complex carbohydrates into the body. Do not forget, then, that proteins are the food from which you take the most energy, the macronutrients that deserve the "superior" title.

And for an avalanche of reasons. In addition to being an essential and therefore fundamental macronutrient for the optimal functioning of our organism, proteins—especially when taken at breakfast and combined with healthy fats and some complex carbohydrates—also boast other extraordinary qualities, including:

- Positive effects on insulin levels, which leads to better consumption of excess fats

- A sense of satiety that fights hunger attacks

- A constant source of energy until noon so that you can forget any sense of tiredness and low motivation

- A fundamental help to improve concentration

- A positive signal to send to your brain as early in the morning, which will make it easier to follow your healthy habits throughout the day

That's why I highly recommend you forget the excuses and theories that are neither in heaven nor on earth that breakfast would be overrated—trust only useful advice!

And it's not like it takes hours and hours to make you breakfast. Check out one of my favorite recipes; you will find it and enjoy it by clicking the link as soon as possible. From breakfast to habit, that in the last period greatly influences my life. An addiction that shuts up destroys a lot of lives; even I have to admit: that's the way it is.

First, I had the feeling that those who warned me of this danger were exaggerating, but then I realized that this was a real problem that puts the lives of many of us at risk. And the most shocking thing is that we don't notice it. So, At this point, I need a dry answer. An increasing number of individuals have fallen into the social media trap. I admit I fell for it, too. As soon as you open your eyes, you are already looking for the latest updates and news on Facebook, Instagram, Twitter, and other sites. This is precisely the move that often, if not always, marks your day.

All that information that, in most cases, has nothing to do with your life confuses your ideas and harms your well-being.

The posts are often orchestrated and show only a small piece of "private life" or just those moments that everyone wants to share with the world, which affects your motivation, concentration, and dedication.

You start to lose touch with real-life easily, and this is reflected, then, on your well-being. Let's face it!

The Task That Marks Your Life

For this reason, I have created for you a mini-challenge with a strong impact on the quality of your daily life.

If you want to change, you have to promise me that for the next 14 days, after hearing the alarm clock, you will not pick up your mobile phone. Take five minutes just for yourself!

And that is sit down, take a few deep breaths, close your eyes, and view your day. Think about your homework, your goals, and your promises, why you're grateful for life, and get ready to start the day peacefully.

I know that not everyone can take up this challenge because they think it is excessive. But those at the game are excited about this very small change and notice a huge difference. That's why I trust you and your decision. In this way, you can:

- Be more positive

- Clarify your thoughts

- Eliminate mood swings

- Stay motivated

- Notice the beautiful things in life that you often ignore

- Be more effective

- Save so much precious time

Once you fall into the social trap, you lose touch with time, so don't take advantage of all those hours when you could do something more concrete. For example, introduce into your life the common habit of those who have no problem leading a healthy lifestyle and who feel good in their own body.

A Few Minutes to Make Your Day Great

A trick related to nutrition, or rather to the organization of meals by meticulously planning your morning activities, you can always find a few precious minutes and prepare one meal—just one, nothing more.

Take less than 10 minutes of your free time to stay on the right track, even during the most critical phase of the day: you will slowly optimize your organizational skills and introduce your body foods that stimulate the consumption of excess fats.

Remember that it is essential to take an excellent source of energy that burns fat residues!

You can do this with a mini snack, that is, a handful of nuts and a few pieces of fruit, you can enjoy a smoothie, take a plastic container and combine some authentic Greek yogurt, berry fruits, and seeds, or you can indulge in some healthy bruschetta.

Long story short: enjoy a healthy, delicious, and balanced snack. I am not talking about specialties worthy of the best chefs globally, but a few simple moves for a completely different day. I guarantee it's worth it! There is, however, also a fourth-morning trick, which in my opinion, is the least frequent but whose potential is spectacular.

Become a Master of Discipline

Especially since it is a morning routine with a strong impact on the discipline, we both know that this is a very important element if you want to make the most of your potential and live your life to the full. And when you wonder why certain people can effortlessly follow the advice and principles of a healthy lifestyle, you'll find a fairly simple answer: they know how to improve this side of their character until they comply with the rules without any problems. Can you do it too? Well, I'm just telling you, today's your lucky day.

The trick with which you will become a real master of discipline is morning physical activity! Don't get me wrong, and I'm not talking about classic workouts that last at least half an hour

I'm talking about a simple task, like:

- Stretching

- A quick walk

- Tabata exercises or other tabata

- Training on stationary bikes or treadmills

So, 10 minutes of one of these activities every day increases self-discipline. Sooner or later, and without much effort, you will find yourself on the right path where nothing can put a spanner in the works anymore. Of course, the results will not be seen immediately.

Don't rush. What matters is to step by step. Already a morning activity twice a week is a nice achievement. If you want to get fairytale results, then you have to follow these wonderful habits and include them in your lifestyle that you will follow without much trouble.

And in the morning, it is ideal to use these tricks, thus creating a solid basis to add the other healthy lifestyle elements.

Don't Forget!

All meals are equally important. I know how hard it is to count every calorie and create recipes based on the optimal macronutrient amount. It took me over six months, but slowly and without thinking too much,

I started doing it automatically and quickly. But you won't need six months. Why not? Because I have created for you a custom menu, depending on your needs.

Food, advice, and tricks: get back in shape without making absurd sacrifices. Would you like to make a diet without making a diet? Would you like to lose weight without moving a finger or have a magic wand and say mysterious formulas to get back in shape?

No serious person or respectable item will ever promise you fast and painless weight loss, but following some tricks and simple rules, you will have excellent results.

10 Good Eating Habits

- Start with the anti-hunger salad; make a small starter made with raw salad, topped with some extra virgin olive oil and lemon, or a yogurt sauce. Do not forget about the mixed seeds (flax, sesame, pumpkin, sunflower) that provide the body with omega 3, 6, and 9 and rich in fiber and antioxidants. The result? You will be less hungry, protect the stomach, and facilitate digestion.

- Replace the sautéed with the broth, vegetables possibly. And use the oil sparingly and always raw.

- Use spices. They are an excellent alternative to salt to flavor your dishes: cumin, turmeric, ginger, nutmeg, cardamom, and fresh aromatic herbs such as thyme, Majorana, sage, and rosemary.

- Choose fast cooking for vegetables. Because the faster it is, the fewer vitamins and mineral salts are lost: prolonged cooking leads to the loss of up to 80% of vitamins.

- Eat products in season and from "natural" crops and farms (without chemical additives or near toxic waste). And especially at zero kilometers, that is, of the area.

- Make small portions and do not give up.

- Eat sugars in the morning; you will get rid of them better.

- Replace alcohol with a fruit cocktail, strictly non-alcoholic. Order the aperitif a "discord" tomato juice (no oil, but with lemon juice and paprika).

- Drink 1.5 liter or 2 liters of water, natural or otherwise hypersonic.

- Let the eyes eat first and then the mouth. That is, it presents well the dishes, color takes care of the choice of raw materials.

10 Easy Habits to Lose Weight Quickly

Don't Skip Meals Anymore

In general, a good rule to make the body give up its kilos too much is not to staff at it, skipping meals or fasting.

But satisfy the sense of hunger.

For this reason, it is very important not to skip meals and eat even between main meals if we feel the need. Our metabolism slows down.

Train Half an Hour a Day

It doesn't take much longer to keep in training, and it's a practical scheme for those short on time.

Half an hour a day every day except one rest, it's a great way to train quickly.

Do you think that's not enough? Train muscle groups at half-time: one day arms and pectorals, the day after belly and legs. All you need is a mat, a chair, or a medical ball, pound weights, and a touch of goodwill.

Prefer Natural Food

Avoid carbonated drinks and any industrial and prepared food, such as biscuits, snacks, ready-made, frozen soups.

Eat Easily

Think about preparing food as easily as possible on the days of the week, reserving one or two more elaborate recipes for Sundays.

Prepare roasted meat and fish with stir-fried vegetables, omelets, salads, simple pasta dishes and vegetables or legumes for lunch, a slice of homemade cake for breakfast.

Metabolism will improve as well as your digestion.

Don't Sit When You Can Stand

Standing, you burn more calories. You only sit when you need to.

Ensure Enough Sleep

At least 7/8 hours of sleep a day improves metabolism and reduces stress, impairs weight loss.

Use Weekends for Rest and Health

Use a few hours on Saturdays and Sundays to prepare weekly meals, for example, by cooking rice or legumes and freezing them, cleaning vegetables, cooking a few dishes in advance. And otherwise, relax.

Ready Meals

Let's say you have little time to cook. Better to make a salad and order a spit chicken than not order a pizza. Today the offer of meals to order in restaurants and rotisseries has expanded a lot, so it is also easy to order (for example, with just eating) complete dishes such as cereals, vegetables, stews, and the usual Chinese or the usual pizza.

Eat More Fiber

It is proven that eating 30-35 grams of fiber per day helps to lose weight.

Make Healthy Snacks

Raw fruit or carrot are great alternatives to bars, snacks, and tramezzini.

Lose Weight Without Upsetting Habits

The Gift diet to lose weight without disrupting eating habits. It is a diet that can cause you to lose up to 3 kg in a week. If you combine it with good and regular physical activity, you can also get a perfect shape. The Gift diet does not cut calories but simply asks you to change the type you eat. It is based on a simple decalogue, flexible, and adaptable to everyone. Every day you must not miss protein foods in the three main meals, fruits and vegetables.

Drink plenty of water, about two liters a day, introduce it with fruits and vegetables rich in it, and take a lot of fiber that optimizes digestive functions. All junk foods are prohibited, even those with preservatives, dyes, flavorings, thickeners, and additives. A psychophysical balance will gradually be achieved, and if you avoid nervous hunger due to stress, nervousness, and other psychological factors, you can lose weight. Help lose weight with a little healthy physical activity, which stimulates metabolism and helps you lose those excess pounds.

But let's see what you eat in a complete weekly menu example.

Monday: Breakfast with a cup of partially skimmed milk, one coffee, one yogurt, two rusks with honey, one boiled egg, one fruit. Snack: 1 apple. Lunch: bresaola with arugula and grana, carrots, boiled zucchini, one sandwich with cooked ham, fruit salad without sugar. Snack: 1 banana. Dinner: 1 slice of swordfish, salad, two slices of wholemeal bread, natural blueberries.

Tuesday: Breakfast with a cup of partially skimmed milk, one coffee, one yogurt with cereals, two slices of bread with cottage cheese, two slices of cooked ham, one para. Snack: 1 apple. Lunch: salad with radicchio, lettuce, tuna, olives, cheese, two slices of bread, fruit salad without sugar Snack: smoothie with one apple, one carrot, and one kiwi. Dinner: fusilli with pesto, apple, and pear mousse.

- **Wednesday:** Breakfast with a cup of green tea, one yogurt with cereals, two wholemeal rusks with honey, one kiwi. Snack, squeezed with one grapefruit and one orange. Lunch, a sandwich with speck, porcini, and radicchio, fruit salad with yogurt. Snack, one banana. Dinner, legume soup with whole-grain croutons, one piece of Parmigiano or provolone, mixed salad, one apple.

- **Thursday:** Breakfast with a cup of partially skimmed milk, a coffee, yogurt with cereals, two wholemeal rusks with honey, one boiled egg, one grapefruit. Snack, two slices of pineapple. Lunch, tagliolini with vegetable ragout, boiled chard, fruit salad without sugar. Snack, one banana. Dinner, roast chicken, baked potatoes, salad, two slices of pineapple.

- **Friday:** Breakfast with a cup of partially skimmed milk, one coffee, yogurt with granola, two slices of bresaola, two wholemeal rusks with sugar-free jam. Snack, one kiwi. Lunch, whole grain Annette with zucchini and shrimp, two boiled eggs, grilled vegetables, fruit salad without sugar. Snack, a smoothie with one apple, one carrot, and one kiwi. Dinner, chickpea soup, mixed salad, two slices of wholemeal bread, and an apple.

- **Saturday:** Breakfast, a cup of partially skimmed milk, one coffee, one yogurt with granules, a small toast with one slice of cooked ham and one slice of fontina, one kiwi. Snack one squeezed grapefruit and one orange. Lunch, octopus and boiled potato salad with celery and carrots, boiled spinach, two slices of pineapple. Snack, a banana. Dinner, trout with paper, baked potatoes, salad, natural berries.

- **Sunday:** Breakfast with a cup of partially skimmed milk, a coffee, yogurt with cereals, one sandwich with jam without sugar, one apple. Snack: a pear. Lunch: lasagna with vegetables, boiled spinach, natural fruit salad. Snack: centrifuged with fresh fruit to taste. Dinner: 1 whole yogurt with hazelnuts, raisins, nuts, pine nuts, almonds, one green apple.

Exercises to Lose Weight Quickly

The feat of losing weight quickly relies on nutrition, but diet alone cannot be a good strategy. It is advisable, and often necessary, constant physical activity, made of daily movement and specific exercises to lose weight: some manage to act more effectively on the body's sensitive points.

A solid daily workout plan can, of course, be made in the gym, thanks to the help of experienced trainers and personal trainers.

But if there is no such possibility, there are several precautions, good habits to build an active lifestyle and exercises to do at home to lose weight, even in the absence of equipment.

In this case, adjust the effort according to your current training condition and fitness: do not submit to the excessive effort, which can hurt you and make the work done to lose weight vain. In this mini-guide, we review the main exercises to promote rapid slimming, from the easiest to the most structured.

Easy Exercises That Burn a Lot of Fat

First of all, there are some basic exercises, practicable every day without any tool. Especially during daily life: constantly "moving" in this way, slimming will be a much faster process than you think. The exercises to devote a specific hour are of great support, but it is even better if they are based on an active and non-sedentary lifestyle.

- Walking, the most "do it yourself" exercise that exists. And, perhaps, for this reason, too often taken for granted or even forgotten: walking even short stretches (such as the way to work, or to accompany children to school) helps a lot, both to lose weight and to maintain an optimal and constant shape over time. If you find yourself walking little for work, a solution for when you are at home is to walk on site.

- To make the stairs is a similar argument to the previous one. If the plans aren't too many, if you don't carry big weights, why not take a little off? The uphill movement, which defies gravity, burns even more fat than the simple path.

- The bicycle, a healthy (and ecological) alternative to walking when the road to do is greater. It puts legs and arms in a great movement, helps to remain toned, and makes you lose weight quickly.

- The step is the continuous ascent and descent from a slight rise, first with one leg and then with the other. These exercises are very simple to do even without the tool since it is enough to practice on a step of the stairs and burn a lot of fat even in a few minutes of training.

Exercises to Quickly Lose Thighs and Buttocks

Some specific workouts act more on the legs' area to make the thighs and buttocks lose weight more quickly. Let's see some examples:

- Lunges exercises are based on the legs' bending, which involves quadriceps and significantly affects the fat accumulated in the thighs and buttocks. The famous squats bend that work similarly.

- Spinning and stationary bike consists of greater effort and is more suitable for athletes. The stationary bike is lighter and, therefore, better for those out of training. These activities consist of high-intensity movements, located mainly in the legs, reducing their fat accumulations.

- The elliptical, a machine available only in the gym, adds an important movement of the arms to the exercise bike's classic action.

- The implant's movements, with firm hands on the hips, in which the leg is raised until it brings the knee to the stomach (to be practiced alternating the two legs).

To effectively lose thighs and buttocks, try a workout based on lunges, squats, exercise bikes, and ellipticals.

Exercises for Belly and Hips

Some other exercises focus more on burning the adipose of the belly and hips. Here are some examples:

- The crunch is a basic exercise for abdominal muscles. It is to be done lying in a supine position, with outstretched arms, with legs joined and flexed at about 90 degrees: these are forward bends, in which only the shoulders are raised. There are several variants.

- The plank, to be done lying on one side: it is resting on the forearm and then lifting the pelvis, keeping the body straight for a few seconds. Afterward, the exercise should be repeated turned on the other side and then with the other arm.

- These-called" bicycle, "lying down, with his arms next to his body and his flying legs, moving just as they were pedaling.

Many of the exercises already described also act importantly on the belly and hips, especially the exercise bike, walks, and corsets.

How to Create and Apply Habits to Lose Weight

A balanced diet and regular physical activity are two fundamental ingredients in the recipe to lose weight healthily and safely. Overweight or obese people usually try different methods of losing weight, intending to improve the silhouette.

They are aware that getting lean would benefit their physical and mental well-being.

Becoming lean is not an easy task, and even if there are different habits useful for this purpose, it is not a goal achieved overnight. Some diets indeed promise miraculous results in a few days, but the best thing is to lose weight gradually without putting your health at risk.

The fact is that, although it is stressful for many people not to see the desired results right away, slimming takes time if you reach the goal healthily and stably.

Fortunately, it is enough to adopt a series of small daily habits to start noticing the first changes, avoiding too rigid or dangerous programs. Today we want to talk to you about the eight best habits so that you can put them into practice right away.

Put Healthier Foods in Plain Sight

Having healthier food insight helps improve your eating habits when you want to lose a few kilos too much.

Arranging fruits and vegetables on the table or even having a handful of dried fruits on hand keeps us away from calorie-rich nibbles, such as fried or sweet foods.

Use Small Plates

It might seem like a stupid thing, but using small plates is very useful when you want to keep track of the number of calories of main meals portions, therefore, are smaller, and since they take up all available space on the plate, the brain senses that they are enough to satiate the appetite.

Increase Fruit and Vegetable Consumption to Become Lean

Daily consumption of five or six servings of raw fruits and vegetables helps promote excess fat elimination. The high water, fiber, and antioxidant compounds stimulate eliminating waste and prevent it from compromising metabolic health.

Also, it brings an important dose of energy to the body, improving its productivity from a mental and physical point of view. What's more, fruits and vegetables prolong the feeling of satiety and reduce the tendency to consume more calories than necessary.

Eat Slowly to Get Lean

Eating voraciously minimizes the secretion of chemicals that generate the feeling of satiety, so you tend to overeat. Although many do it unconsciously, it is necessary to improve this habit to prevent it from negatively affecting weight.

Taking enough time to eat calmly allows you to chew foods better and avoids exceeding calories.

Drink Water and Healthy Drinks

Increasing water and healthy drinks is a great way to promote metabolism and weight loss's proper functioning.

Liquids moisturize the body's cells, improve the purification process of excretory organs, and help maintain the feeling of satiety for longer.

Depuratively owned teas, green smoothies, and fruit-flavored waters are great options to include in slimming diets.

Sleep Well

People who want to lose weight must 100% improve the quality of their rest. It is crucial to achieving good results.

During rest, important functions are activated for metabolism and, as a result, the production of hormones that control hunger increases. Staying awake too long or interrupting sleep increases night cravings and the risk of obesity.

Do Combined Physical Activity to Get Lean

Carrying out cardiovascular physical activity every day is a good way to increase energy consumption and burn fat more easily. If you combine it with strength training, the benefits of losing weight are greater.

Add Toppings to Dishes

The addition of some condiments serves to stimulate the metabolism's functioning to lose the kilos too much.

Spices such as Cayenne chili and turmeric stimulate metabolic activity, improving the transformation of fats into energy. As you have seen, adopting simple habits that help reduce weight, control anxious hunger, and stimulate metabolism is a question. Try to put them into practice right away to complete your food program.

Good Habits That Help You Lose Weight

Drinking and doing physical activity is the basis, but what are the other secrets to losing weight quickly?

We would all like to wake up one morning and magically lose the extra kilos. Unfortunately, it never happens like this. To get back in shape, you need discipline.

Here are ten tips to lose the pounds accumulated from the holidays in a short time.

- Drink only water and at least 2 liters per day

- Do at least 30 minutes of cardio activity per day.

- Drink coffee one hour before training.

- Eliminate carbohydrates or reduce them considerably.

- Make three series of 12 push-ups and squats.

- Sleep at least 30 minutes more.

- Remember to drink warm water and lemon to make detox.

- It is recommended to eat less and lighter in the evening.

- Stay straight. Posture is key.

- Remember to eat fennel and cucumbers in quantity. They have drained and deflating power.

Tips for Slimming Once and for All

Losing weight is difficult, but it is not taking it back can be even more challenging. If you've ever regained weight after losing it, getting on a scale fills you with worry.

The happiness you feel when you reach your shape weight can be completely erased and replaced by frustration, confusion, and sadness when you pick up the weight you lost. But you're not alone—whether it's your metabolism that's problematic, that you struggle to eat healthily or do regular physical activity, whether it's the drugs that make you gain weight, know that many people struggle with this same problem. Thankfully there are effective ways to lose weight once and for all.

While there isn't a trick that works for everyone, these ten tips for permanently losing weight will help you maintain the shape weight you've conquered with so much effort.

Do Regular Physical Activity and Vary Exercises

Physical activity is a key element in losing extra pounds. Many people fight to lose weight even if they do physical activity regularly due to how they exercise.

The fact is that following an exercise routine is not the best or most effective way to lose weight permanently. Because? Even if you lose some weight and maybe manage to keep your new weight shape for a while, doing the same exercises every day doesn't give you all the benefits that physical activity could provide you if you changed your exercise routine frequently or tried something completely new. To put it simply, make your muscles work and strengthen more if you add a little variety.

Often, you get bored always to follow the same exercise routine, and many people end up skipping the gym or no longer training at home just out of boredness.

This phenomenon is very common, especially when the mood is affected by colder temperatures and when the days get shorter. To prevent it from happening, sign up for a new course or start training for a race before getting bored.

Say No

There's nothing worse than the guilt you feel when someone cooks something just for you. These are usually delicious cookies, cakes, or sweets—things that you probably have to avoid if you follow a diet and that aren't healthy food choices anyway. And it's always fun (or annoying) when someone cooks for you but doesn't want to eat a portion of the cake too. These people pushing you to eat can be hard to handle if you don't want to be rude or make you think you don't appreciate their effort.

Although the thought is kind, it can push some people to let go of healthy food choices. For those who have struggled to lose weight and are fighting to stay in their weight, these challenges offered are a temptation that you would not want to have to face regularly. Almost everyone struggles to say no, and so they often give themselves more than they would like. The best thing to do is to say no and explain that you are trying to eat healthy even if you appreciate the thought. In this way, it is hoped the person in question will not repeat the same error. Enjoy a piece of cake now and then if you want, but let others take the leftovers home if they wish.

Engage Family and Friends

One step beyond the art of saying no is the involvement of the people you spend the most time with within your healthy lifestyle—try to make everyone understand your new healthy habits and to respect them. The people around you can both help you and put your health goals at risk.

Share your goals with them and explain how you intend to achieve them. A support network can motivate you a lot, but most importantly, you'll avoid being regularly tempted to break your new rules.

If you have a family, engage in your weight loss strategy by planning tasks to do together to stay active. When it's cold, pack up and go hiking or spend the day in the snow in winter. If you go to the beach, bring a soccer or volleyball ball instead of sunbathing all day. In large groups of family or friends, organize a friendly (or competitive if you prefer) match of your favorite sport.

Weighed Regularly

You may need to try several times to determine how long to weigh yourself, but you'll find the ideal frequency that allows you to stay focused on your slimming goals. Start getting on the scale every week or every two weeks and see how it makes you feel. Weighing yourself regularly can help you and motivate you to eat better and exercise as you'll have to account for the scales.

It is important to note that several factors can cause fluctuations in body weight, which depend on the diet you follow, sex, the time of day you weigh yourself, and how much physical activity you do. It's very common for women to have weight fluctuations of up to a kilo a day, so don't get scared and don't get demoralized. If you are gaining weight regularly, it starts to weigh you every day or one day yes and one day not, and take into account your eating habits and physical activity to understand what can be the cause of weight gain. After analyzing your habits, if you cannot locate this cause, talk to a doctor about it because some diseases and drugs can cause weight gain.

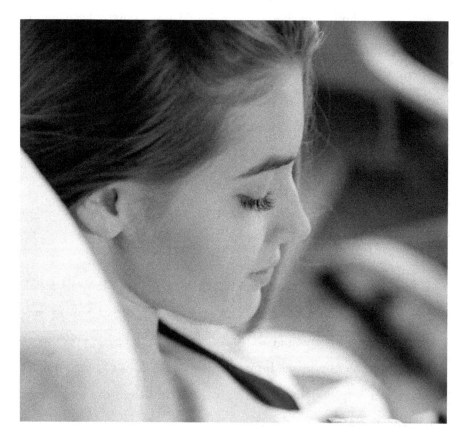

Find a Diet Companion

One of the easiest ways not to regain weight is to have someone who has similar goals. It can be a friend or family member, or even someone you met in the gym. No matter who it is, there's nothing like supporting and understanding someone who's going through the same problems as you.

This type of relationship can also provide you with the motivation and encouragement you need to follow your new healthy lifestyle. Check that the person you have in mind has a positive attitude because someone who always complains and has a negative attitude can become an obstacle to your efforts.

A diet companion can help you in many ways, as well as support you emotionally and mentally. The relationship's social dimension gives you something positive to wait for during a hard day's work or a stressful period.

Your companion can also give you the self-confidence you need to try something new. It could be a simple thing, like enrolling in a new course you didn't want to attend on your own, or something more challenging than starting training for a race.

Stay Focused Even After Reaching the Goal

One of the easiest and fastest ways to regain lost weight is to stop doing what helped you reach your weight shape. It should come as no surprise to regain weight when you stop eating well and doing physical activity. Your body loses fat and weight, especially by following a healthy diet, strengthening and toning muscles, and regularly doing cardiovascular activities. If you stop following these healthy habits, the extra kilos come back very soon!

Another situation that causes the recovery of weight loss after significant weight loss is drastic diets. Millions of people follow drastic diets to lose weight quickly, only to be frustrated when the weight comes back shortly after the diet. This often happens with diets cutting out of feeding entire food groups. You start eating what you cut off from the diet for a while, and the extra pounds are back there, along with inches of the thigh. Instead of doing drastic diets, follow a healthy diet, and have regular physical activity to lose weight. If you eliminate a food group from your diet, you will not get any results if you want to start eating those same foods again. So just don't do it.

Follow a Healthy and Balanced Lifestyle

Many people try to lose weight by doing only one thing: eating healthy or doing physical activity. Doing just one of two things can help you lose weight, and you might as well achieve your goals, but the best way to make it last is to live a healthy and balanced lifestyle that includes both a healthy diet and regular exercise.

Eating foods low in harmful fats, sugars, and sodium can help you lose weight quickly if you now eat many unhealthy foods or have bad eating habits. But you will have achieved the first goal when eating healthy will no longer be enough to make you lose weight. Lack of regular exercise can increase the risk of even serious illnesses and complications, so try to eat well and exercise to get the maximum benefits and not bring back the extra pounds you've lost. Conversely, by doing some physical activity but continuing to eat unhealthy foods, you may lose weight. Still, without eliminating the dangers of poor nutrition—even the fittest people risk having health problems due to a bad diet.

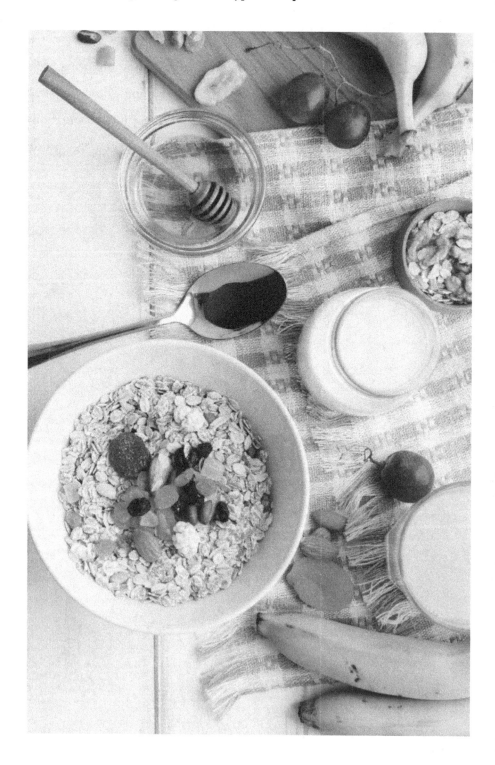

Chapter 2.

How to Create New Habits

A lifestyle change—whether it is you want to lose weight, improve in sports, increase well-being—implies creating new habits.

Otherwise, you have only a mediocre and temporary result. In this section, we find out how to build habits. But first of all:

Habit

A habit is a collection of behaviors and abilities. It is a series of steps, made without mental commitment because that series has already been repeated several times: it has been learned.

A habit can be small, such as drinking a little bit of water (hence the famous saying, "It's as simple as"), or very complicated, like putting together what you need to build a website or start a Fitness journey.

In creating a habit, it is essential to have the ability to learn the skills necessary to do so. You can't build a website if you don't know what the Internet is, and you can't start a Fitness path if you don't know what fitness is! Don't believe everything, a lot of people don't know.

How to Build a Habit

Once you have chosen habits or skills to develop, you need to figure out how to precede them to develop them. It can be applied in Fitness and any other sector where there is a need to "learn progressively" (What is the area where there is no such need?).

Search for Templates and Guides

Watching and interacting with others is the way we humans have to learn. Behaviors, abilities, and habits do not passively absorb them from others, but at all times, we decide what we want to learn and what we want to discard. We do this based on the goals we want to achieve ("What I want to achieve") and the values we want to have ("What characterizes me").

Pro-actively observing others (asking questions where needed) is the best way to learn new habits.

Taking Small Steps

To create a new habit or skill and include it in your life, it is important to take small steps at a time (adjusting the frequency with which to do them properly).

For example, if you are not a marathon runner, it is unthinkable to start a training program that uses marathon runners for several years. Small steps may seem trivial and non-goal-oriented. Inquiring about the best running shoes, knowing if you are physically suitable, and so on are those fundamental "small steps" to create new habits.

In essence, the first step in building good habits is to learn what steps should be taken: learning the steps to take (planning) is part of learning the new habit. Cognitive Psychology studies, by the way, teach us this: the time is taken to plan, and the time taken to act is inversely proportional. Those who invest little time in planning lose a lot in the action phase. With the difference that more wrong actions lead to frustration, decreased self-esteem, poor motivation.

Persist

"If you commit to something, you eventually get a certain result." In short: it is not possible that if you commit to something, in the end, you do not get "anything."

Often, especially when it comes to weight loss, it is thought that a diet or training to lose weight has not produced results. It is thought that nothing has "changed." But this reasoning is deleterious. It only looks at the visible effect. Rather than get frustrated and get stuck, you should ask yourself: If my body hasn't changed, what else has changed? Or What inhibited the change in my body?

In short, if you learn to evaluate your fitness level true and deep (for this, we recommend that you do it by familiarizing with our method here), not only by persisting you will approach the goals you want to achieve, but you will also appreciate aspects that you previously thought were "collateral."

Avoid hyper-enthusiastic attitudes typical of those who start "bombshell" with a new diet, training, program, complex and detailed, and then give up exhausted after a short time. In the first 1-2 months of a new approach, a new diet, a new workout, a new program, everything seems easy.

But be aware of motivation: it's a double-edged sword. Motivation allows you to turn on the engines and push yourself into the open sea, but habits allow you to continue sailing and arriving at your destination.

And building a habit takes perseverance in those 1-2 months, focusing on simple little actions even though you would have the motivation to do more complicated and advanced things at that moment.

At first, you will need some effort. Over time, the mental load will decrease, and those actions will become habits. At this point, you can enter other actions, other details, which will make you create a new habit.

Be Aware

Repetition is essential to develop new skills and create a new habit (or multiple habits). But repeating them without awareness does not favor memorization. It ends that, the moment you have to repeat that action, you will be forced to "re-enter into practice." Think of the "strokes of luck" or the "fortune of the beginner": textbook actions that come out randomly and precisely fortuitous.

We would all like to repeat those actions in the same way, but we cannot because we have not repeated them, but we have not been aware of the key steps.

In consolidating a habit and make it so, it is necessary to be aware of every step taken and study every detail and go out again to observe the general picture and understand how everything is cohesive. Otherwise, you risk being overwhelmed: you can't remember every detail.

Think, for example, if for every healthy meal, you should remember how to build the meal itself from macronutrients and calories or a workout starting with exercises, series, and repetitions. It is necessary to find the general scheme that allows you to reconstruct, at all times, and "to the need"—without having to keep everything in memory, constantly—the various details.

Stay Motivated by Looking Into Perspective

It happens to everyone to have moments where they say, "Who made me do it?" to look at that caramel cheesecake and think, "Why am I here too fast?" to go to the gym with the fear of fatigue that will be felt in training. That's normal. More: it's physiological.

In these cases, it is advisable to look into perspective. Since it is difficult to do so "in those moments," it would be useful to have written previously (or to have strongly consolidated in your memory) what your long-term mission is.

There are times when it seems to us that some of the choices made were at odds with our mission when we had already evaluated them at the table.

Simply, the moment we put them into practice, we said, "But why am I doing this?". Go back to the paragraph above (Persist) to answer this question.

"Pay pledge" (subject to reservation) It might be useful to declare (to others or yourself, for example, on your diary/logbook) that you want to create a new habit. "I want to eat healthily," "I want to go to bed early," "I want to exercise at least two times a week," "I want to be able to drink eight glasses of water a day," and so on. Declaring this could be useful because, for consistency, there will be a tendency to respect this.

But watch out. In this way, the motivation could move from internal to external, losing the sense of what you want to do: you could risk doing something just because "you are following the pattern"

If you do not follow it, you will have to "pay pledge." To avoid this, from time to time (for example, every 30 days), check/update what you have stated, reorganizing your action plan based on new needs and (possibly) new goals.

Swing Around Your Balance

Unfortunately, many "Mind Professionals" (all those who deal with the mind and psyche, such as Psychologists, Mind Coaches, and others) seem to strongly beat only on creating good habits in the long run. As if only the first part of this article existed.

But it is essential to understand that the human being also needs to satisfy momentary pleasures.

It is peremptory to insert breaks from positive habits within a path to create a new habit (or more habits). Are you trying to create the new habit of studying a new language for at least an hour a day? Take one day of the week when you don't think about it.

In creating a new habit, you should always ensure a break that satisfies a momentary pleasure, even if opposed to what you want to achieve in the long term.

If you think about it, the action is opposed, but it allows the new habit to consolidate faster, relieving the required cognitive commitment. In the diet: insert a delicious, at first also daily, small, then weekly; every 2-4 months enter 1-2 weeks softer. In training: For each workout, include a part (10-20% of the training time, for example) to have fun; or, a workout of the week, dedicate it to completely different exercises or activities.

About the "mindset": When joining your plan/route, set a day when you live without a port at all what your goal is. Think of any other factor and, within the process of creating a new habit, enter the corresponding "non-habit" (that is, what contrasts with the one you want to build).

Do not seek balance, but a healthy oscillation around your equilibrium point.

Habits That Build Habits

We are human beings: our cognitive abilities are mind-blowing, but our ability to allocate resources (energy, land-to-earth: sugar/ATP) to them is ridiculous. Whether you want it or not, the brain has limited energy to allocate to various cognitive processes.

The blanket is always short: if you put on one side, remove it from another.

If you are trying to create a new habit, such as "Brushing your teeth three times a day by staying at least 3 minutes", it will be more difficult to do so with a sleep deficit on your shoulders.

Therefore, it will be useful to create a new habit—for example—"Sleep at least 7 hours a day going to bed by 23:00".

Simply because cognitive energy is not "spiritual" energy, but concrete: energy used by the brain in the form of glucose/ATP/other energy substrates, which are not indefinite, that's why habits—all habits—have these characteristics:

A habit can "activate" another habit. For example: if a person wants to exercise in the morning (because he can't remember the rest of the day), he has to wake up early and wake up early. He has to go to bed early. In that case, the habit of going to bed early "activates" the habit of exercising in the morning.

A habit can "allow" another habit. The same example: if you want to exercise (in the morning as at another time of the day), and you are sleepy because you sleep little, exercise will not be so pleasant (and therefore you will not have the motivation to repeat it). In that case, the habit of going to bed early "allows" the habit of exercising.

Next, here are some habits without which creating a new habit will be impossible. You can define them as the basic habits to create a new habit.

Sleeping Well

There is no precise amount of hours: the average is between 7 and 9 hours a day, but everyone should find their own. If you can, waking up without a wake-up call allows it: the first few days, you will probably sleep more; but then you will stick to your rhythm. Instead, if you use the alarm clock, use one as a Sleep Cycle, which wakes up at the most propitious moment (within a preset range).

Don't eat "too well." The title of the paragraph is not advising you to eat little, but not to magic "too well": fall into the obsession of clean foods, of following the diet, counting calories, you do not need it. You need to learn to eat healthy foods, in such quantities that you do not feel "restricted" (the important thing is not to get engulfed with every meal).

Or, rather, don't feel like you're on a diet. Find out how to make a "non-diet" here.

Body Hygiene

Washing your hands, teeth, and having the feeling of constant freshness, predisposes to a positive mood that allows you to face better new commitments (such as creating a new habit). Do not neglect these small factors. They can change your day.

Exercise Breathing and Stretching

"Training" is one count, but you can't do training without the basics to master your body. Dedicating yourself to breathing awareness, making light stretching, and improving posture come before any training (on pain of poor results, not commensurate with the effort spent).

Learning to Relax

There is no need to do Yoga or, better, doing Yoga should not mean being a conservationist. It only takes a few minutes and a couple of exercises to learn to relax. Not only that: a walk on the sea at sunset or sunrise, listening to music, being outdoors are also "techniques" to relax.

Stay Connected (Not Technology!)

The connection with others and with Nature is fundamental—it is one of the universal needs of the human being who, if not satisfied, can give rise to abnormal behaviors.

Sticking to your smartphone on every occasion when "nothing is being done" (which could be exploited simply to make yourself aware of your breath or look at the landscape outside) kills self-awareness, libido, and creativity.

Lose Weight Fast and Naturally

You're tired of miracle diets that don't help you lose weight. Your almost daily visit to the gym doesn't make you lose weight at the rate you would like. Don't despair.

You may have to, as the Anglo-Saxons say, "go back to basics" and start opting for less complicated and more natural solutions.

To do this, and being already in the middle of summer, the idea is to "take advantage" of the resources and opportunities that the warmest season of the year gives us.

The All for Fashion Design website suggests a series of practices that are easy to carry out during the summer and that can, with some constancy, help us lose weight.

The importance of green tea. Green tea is one of the best drinks to lose weight quickly. It is recommended to drink four to five cups of green tea a day for good results.

Much of its success is due to catechin. This antioxidant owns this plant, which helps our body increase cellular metabolism and, consequently, burn fats more quickly and effectively.

Good Tricks to Lose Weight in Summer

Water and more water: Start the morning drinking water and keep it up all day long. Its refreshing and satiating power will help you cope with the high temperatures and not exceed the beach's meals.

They are easy and available ways for anyone to lose weight in summer. In addition to keeping the body hydrated, drinking water helps burn calories and keeps your metabolism in great condition, so don't waste the opportunity to drink a glass of the liquid element from time to time.

- **Outdoor training:** When we're not on alert for heatwaves, it's not a bad idea to replace the gym with some outdoor activity. Running, playing a football or basketball game, or practicing yoga or aerobic exercises will help you keep your mind and body healthy, help you lose weight, and at the same time, have fun.

- **Laugh a lot:** Summer and holidays are the best scenarios to try to forget or at least park all your problems. So, enjoy the summer and laugh a lot, because, apart from the facial exercise you carry out, various studies show that laughter and lack of stress can lose weight. Take advantage of visits to the beach or the pool to make a few long swimming will not only make your summer more fun but also help you keep your body well-formed and healthy. Swimming reduces the risk of heart disease and helps burn calories.

- **Eat watermelon:** One of the star fruits of summer. The watermelon is delicious, fresh, rich in water, and collaborates crucially in weight loss for its satiating power. Replace calorie meals with a salad. Summer heat makes it more appetizing to replace healthy, fat foods with vitamin-rich vegetables and salads. Your body will thank you.

Energy for the Whole Day

- Water with lemon to wake up. As you can see, we are very much a fan of water. Although now we propose a small alternative: start the day with warm water flavored with lemon. Lemon contains a whole day of vitamin C, a vitamin that lowers cortisol level, which triggers hunger and fat storage.

- Some of the simplest formulas for weight loss are the most effective. Oatmeal, the champions' and perfect breakfast, is here. Prepare a plate of "overnight oats" or oatmeal soaked (see recipe) at night, and by the next day, you'll have it ready. It is rich in fiber and will keep you active throughout the day.

- Sleep is the best fuel. Even though high temperatures are the worst enemy of sleep, you must make sure you can sleep at least 8 hours. Thus, you will wake up with more energy in the morning, which will allow you to face the day with maximum energy.

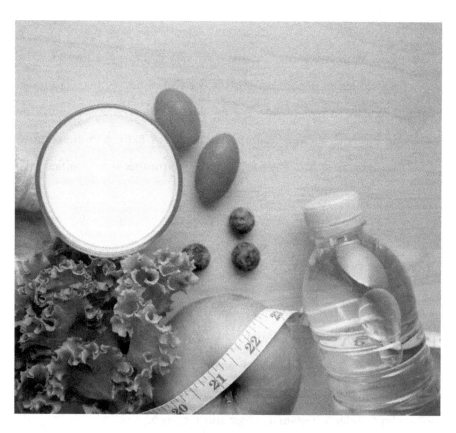

6 Drinks to Lose Weight and Start Losing Weight

100% natural weight loss drink recipes that you can prepare in less than 5 minutes. With them, you will manage to burn fat faster, and you will feel better. If you are thinking of losing weight, you should know that you can lose weight with homemade and natural drinks and follow a diet. With them, you can lose up to five kilos in a week.

We show you several recipes of weight-loss drinks that you can prepare at home before the arrival of summer. Because we are what we eat, and it is best to feed yourself healthily with all that nature offers us. Also, the juice recipes for weight loss are very easy to prepare.

First of all, you must understand that there are no magic solutions, but a healthy and nutrient-rich diet will make us well and in harmony with our body. These are the most effective fat loss juices, but don't forget to exercise regularly and drink two water liters a day.

Coconut Water Juice

It is a very low-calorie drink and has abundant electrolytes; this benefits your nervous system and calms anxiety. It moisturizes you and not only helps you lose weight but helps your metabolism and keeps your skin fresh. Although they sell it prepared, it usually brings added sugar, so we recommend that you buy the coconut and take the natural juice from inside.

Green Tea

This tea is more effective if you take it cold, it can also help you not get cold. Green tea helps metabolism lose fat quickly and effectively, much more than any commercial drink.

Lettuce, Spinach, and Kiwi Juice

To make this simple juice, place in a blender a kiwi, two or three lettuce leaves, and two spinach leaves. Add cold water to thicken, and you can sweeten it with some fruit. It is a drink to lose weight highly recommended and refreshing for summer. This antioxidant drink will also give you an extra energy supply thanks to the vitamin C and chlorophyll it contains.

Grapefruit Juice

Grapefruits are easy to get and are very economical. By taking a single glass of this juice a day, you'll burn all the excess fat, and you'll be able to lose weight easily and quickly. It is recommended that you take it fasting to enhance its effects.

Jamaican Water

To make this drink, you have to buy the Jamaican flowers and boil them for five minutes. It has diuretic properties, so it will help you lose fat without realizing it. You can have up to three glasses a day if you want.

Ginger Tea

Ginger tea wipes out all the accumulated fat, and it does so effectively and naturally. It will also be of great help if you have any breathing problems.

But be careful, you won't be able to drink this drink if you suffer from high blood pressure.

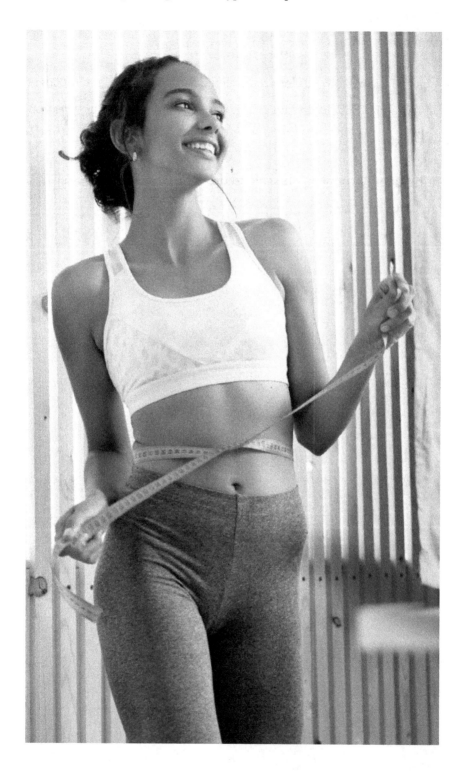

Chapter 3.

Removing the Temptations That Provoke Binges

How to Overcome the Temptation to Eat Foods You Fancy but Fatten

Whether for aesthetic reasons or for some health condition, such as when your doctor tells you to choose low-fat foods or don't add salt to meals, anyone who cares about healthy eating or wants to lose weight will have to overcome the temptation to eat some foods and dishes they want.

This can be a difficult task, so here are some recommendations to reinforce your motivation and not get carried away with cravings.

What a big paradox! The same foods you find delicious are usually just the first foods you have to remove when you're on a diet (for weight loss or other health reasons). They even get tastier and greedy as you know you should avoid eating them, don't you?

Now, what if I told you that the exquisiteness of that delicacy that is melting imaginary between your teeth is cultural or part of your customs? Some studies show that you generally want what you're used to eating. For example, if you replace meat burgers with the same soy product, the former may no longer be so attractive to you after a while, and you may no longer want them so intensely.

Even after a while, you may not like them or feel heavy after eating them.

However, it is true that maintaining motivation and overcoming temptation can be a very difficult task, which has to do not only with your habits but also with your mood and the context around you.

You may even find it impossible to avoid temptation if you participate in meetings and parties constantly or if you have any concerns at work or are anxious for some personal reason.

In short: when it comes to eating and assembling the day's menu, many factors come into play. So, because your concern is to eat a healthy diet and be able to meet your goal without falling into temptation, here are several recommendations that can give you the motivation you need to help you remove from your mind those uncontrollable desires to eat what you shouldn't:

Clear as Water

Every time you're tempted, drink one or two glasses of water. That will make you feel satisfied and alleviate your desires. If the water is not enough, try accompanying it by eating an ounce or 30 grams of nuts (six nuts, 12 almonds, or 20 peanuts).

Free Yourself!

Remove from your cupboard or refrigerator (cooler) those products that you should not eat, so it will be easier for you to avoid them. If you buy them anyway and start feeling guilty while you're eating them, destroy them, throw them away, break them, soak them in water, or do whatever makes you feel better!

Imagine

The temptation may go away if you imagine eating what you so desire when, in fact, what's in your mouth is a healthy thing. Another option is to think of landscapes and even different aromas to divert your mind to other sensations.

Move

Before you go to the cupboard or refrigerator looking for what you want so much, go for a run or walk, jump, go up and down the stairs of the building or do some kind of exercise. By the way, you might lose weight faster.

Get Distracted

If jumping alone in the office bathroom doesn't work, look for some way to distract your mind. For example, you can call a friend, listen to music, or do some errands.

Relax

Stress and tensions can attack your goodwill and make you fall into temptation. Learn how to control your nerves (you can help yourself with relaxation, breathing, meditation, or visualization techniques, for example).

Rest

Fatigue and tiredness can also make you want to eat more. Try to get a good night's sleep and, if you can, it's not enough for you to take a short nap to get your energy back.

Change

Sometimes it can be helpful for you to modify your routines. For example, if you're used to walking in front of a bakery that sells irresistible treats, choose another path and avoid passing by. Other changes? Instead of eating a candy bar or candy, you can sip coffee with skim milk or brush your teeth and gargle, to change the taste of your mouth and make the temptation go away.

Treat Yourself!

Always avoid foods you want so much can ruin your diet when you no longer resist temptation. Once or twice a month, let yourself eat what you love so much, but try to take a small portion.

The important thing is not that you stop eating everything you like or that you repress yourself in front of every bite you want to bring to your mouth. On the contrary, the idea is that you learn to distinguish between foods that are more or less healthy and most appropriate for you.

Cheer Up

Motivation and thinking about food, food, and diet are very important for success. If you stop thinking of certain foods as forbidden and change the way you feed in general by expanding your menu, you will see that it can even become a fun process of discoveries, new aromas, flavors, and why not? Even from family and friends' reactions, you want to surprise with a healthy and equally exquisite menu. Take the test, and then you tell us.

Tips to Avoid Compulsive Eating and Binge Eating

Did you know that compulsive eating and bingeing are among the most common eating disorders in the United States? (Source: NCBI) It's such a common eating disorder that many people have it and don't realize it. Some of us think there's something wrong with us, or we eat like that because we don't have willpower. But there's so much more behind this eating disorder, and there are ways to heal it and avoid falling back into it.

What Compulsive Eating or Binge Eating Is

The official name for this eating disorder is Binge-twisting and involves compulsive eating or consuming abnormal amounts of food while feeling like you can't stop or feel out of control.

Having binges is a period where you can't control the way you eat. You usually eat quickly, passing the point where the individual feels satisfied. Usually, people who have this type of disorder eat due to stress and usually consume large amounts of junk or ultra-processed food, high fat, starches, and calories.

Unfortunately, broccoli or tofu does not cause the same chemical response in our brains, so we always tend to resort to carbohydrates and those that affect brain chemistry.

As you can imagine, compulsive eating can lead to serious health problems.

In addition to being overweight, it can become an excessive weight and generates many other diseases, such as diabetes, heart disease, strokes, certain types of cancer, and more.

In addition to the physical effect that this can generate, compulsive eating also generates a mental and emotional effect.

After losing control over food and overeating, the individual ends up feeling out of control, without any power, and with emotions of grief, depression, and shame.

Symptoms of Compulsive Eating

We've all eaten too much, but if you see that you're often eating out of control or have to eat a lot more in certain situations, such as when you're stressed, then you may need to read the following.

When I used to diet, especially those that were very restrictive, I used to eat compulsively, especially bread, cakes, or carbohydrates that will cross me. As you'll see later on, constant dieting and removing food groups from your diet (usually carbohydrates or fats), you tend to want those "forbidden" foods more. This is part of the natural response from your body and a side effect of dieting.

Behavioral Symptoms

- You can't stop eating, or you can't control what you eat

- Quickly eat large amounts of food

- Eating even when you're already full

- Hide or gather food in a place to eat afterward

- Eat normally or limit yourself when you eat with other people, but eat too much when you're alone

- Eat continuously during the day, without following any eating plans (i.e., without meal hours)

Emotional Symptoms

- Feeling stressed or worried and knowing that just eating relieves these kinds of emotions

- Be ashamed of what you eat and how much

- Feeling unconscious when you're having a binge like you're on autopilot

- Never feel satisfied, no matter how much food you eat.

- Feeling guilty, embarrassed, or depressed after having a binge

- Feel desperate to control weight or lose weight and have very strict rules regarding eating habits.

- You suffer from binge eating disorder

- You are feeling out of control when you eat

- Do you think about food all the time?

- Do you eat in secret?

- Do you eat even when you're already full to the extent that you feel bad?

- Do you eat to manage your emotional needs, such as when you feel stressed, worried, or like to comfort yourself?

- Do you feel sorry or shame after eating?

- Do you feel like you can't control when you stop eating, even if you want to?

The greater the number of affirmations and affirmative answers, the chances are you'll have this type of disorder.

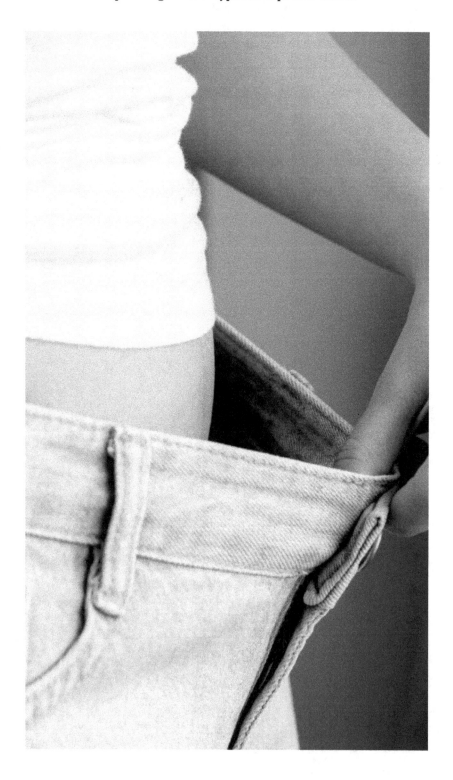

Chapter 4.

The 5 Traps You Should Set to Avoid Eating for Anxiety

Effective tricks to combat anxiety are clear and easy, but you have to follow them to the letter. Cleaning your fridge with temptations and avoiding spending too many hours without taking food are some of them.

We often eat for reasons with little to do with hunger—namely, boredom, sadness, loneliness, or Anxiety. When we eat dominated by emotions, we almost always give ourselves binges caused by cortisol, the stress hormone that triggers the appetite of foods high in fats and sugars. That's what the body asks of us when we're anxious.

To avoid this, you have to put some traps in the path of the binge. It is even worth self-defiance and seeks reward somewhere away from the fridge.

Clean The "Dangerous" Food Fridge

It's not carrot and broccoli that we're going to eat if we're anxious. The normal thing is that we threw something sweet, greasy, with a lot of calories. But if you've previously taken care of cleaning your tempting fridge, you'll be able to get around the time of the binge danger. You'll have to settle for yogurt, a boiled egg, or some fruit. Anything but a cookie, I pray.

Eat at Regular Intervals

The longer you've gone without eating, the more you'll eat. This maxim is almost universal, whether you're anxious or not. It is better to avoid many hours between meals, so you don't eat them all in one go. The idea is to be satisfied and not see food as a reward.

Pay Attention While Eating

This will help you reduce the emotional burden you relate to food. It will also help you chew slower. It is recommended to leave the fork on the table every two bites to slow down the speed at which we usually devour food.

Create a "Safe" Eating Environment

That means not eating in front of the TV or the computer. Also, do not put a full fountain on the table. Serve yourself what you're going to eat on your plate and store the rest in the fridge, so you'll avoid the temptation to repeat.

Change the Hunger Route

If you're nervous, don't always do what you usually do in those cases; avoid going through your favorite junk food restaurant and ordering a burger for dinner at home. Sometimes it works to change activity or take the dog for a walk. On the way back, you won't remember you would pay homage in front of the fridge anymore.

Guide to Eliminating Cravings for Sugar and Processed Food

Different tools to get rid of those cravings for sugar and processed food.

When we talk about "cravings," we mean an intense desire to consume a specific food. It is usually directed towards processed food, which is very tasty because of its high sugar, flours, fat, salt, and additives.

The craving for these meals (also known as ultra-processed) is a multidimensional experience, as it includes cognitive aspects (e.g., thinking a lot about that meal), emotional (the desire to eat or even changes in your mood), behavioral (search, hide, consume that product) and physiological (e.g., salivation).

Since we live in an environment full of ultra-processed products, cravings are very common. More than 50% of people experience cravings regularly (study), and this fact plays a very important role in increasing body fat, "food addiction." The binging that the population has (study). It's emotional eating that can, over time, affect your health.

Realfooder, today I bring you a complete guide to eliminating those cravings based on scientific evidence and my clinical experience. With it, you'll be the one who controls the food and not the food that controls you.

Avoid temptations, ultra-processed away from home. We have a system in our brain, known as the reward system. This system was designed to "reward us" when we do things that improve our survival.

This includes primitive behaviors such as eating, moving, having sex, etc. When we eat, our brain knows that we are doing something "right," and it releases quite a few chemicals, such as the neurotransmitter dopamine that gives us pleasure.

The problem with processed food is that it can cause a much more powerful reward than real food, and that's why generating a dependency where it's useless to say "eat sparingly."

Simply observing or knowing that there are tasty ultra-processed things in our fridge or pantry will trigger the brain to throw a "hook" at us.

Once we experience this desire, there will be a "debate" within us between the pros and cons of eating this processing. We can win that dispute from time to time and resist that sweet bite, but our instinct usually beats us out of perseverance.

Moreover, we do not always have all the "defenses" available to win that debate, sometimes we are bored, stressed, or depressed, and the pros to give us that pleasant moment win by a goal.

If processed products (sweets, baubles, biscuits, pastries, etc.) are not found at home, temptation, and anxiety about eating them are reduced. Maybe the stimulus is so strong it even makes us leave the house. If so, at least we'll buy more time for our minds to discuss whether we really need to eat that processing (and by the way, maybe we'll even move a little).

The problem with removing temptations is that it's not always that easy. We usually live in the company and may not agree with your decision to be a real folder.

You may also be at work, and both in the cafeteria and in the vending machines you have processed or on the street, numerous fast food establishments ask you for a claim. That's why we're going to keep giving tools.

Sleep Better and Manage Stress

Hunger and satiety are affected by hormonal fluctuations throughout the day. Sleep deprivation alters these hormonal signals and can lead to cravings' most common onset. This thesis is supported by a meta-analysis of studies, which shows that people with poor sleep are up to 55% more likely to be obese than people who get enough sleep.

For this reason, before evaluating other factors, we need to assess whether we are resting well on quantity and quality of sleep, whether we are dedicating the attention, time and importance it has in our lives.

Plan your evening tasks well, set the alarm 30 minutes before bedtime, and read a good book (avoid TV light, mobile, iPad). Some magnesium supplements and melatonin can help the most insomniac person.

Also, poor rest can lead to higher levels of stress. We know that stressed people often report having more cravings than non-stressed individuals.

Stress is an ally of cravings for ultra-processed, and studies tell us that even more for women. This study observed how women with high cortisol levels experienced large cravings for stressed processed food than non-stressed ones. Do you know a good natural de-stressor? Exercise.

On numerous occasions, our bodies confuse thirst for some hunger. When we suddenly crave specific processing, try drinking a large glass of water and waiting a few minutes.

It is possible that once calmed, and the thirst also disappears the intensity of the craving.

In general, being well-hydrated benefits people who want to lose weight, but keep an eye on it without performing hyper-hydration follies. In adults, drinking water before meals (250-500 ml) can reduce appetite and weight loss.

Eating Real Food vs. Ultra-Processed Food

The more processed meals you eat, the more cravings you'll have for them. The more real food you eat, the fewer cravings you'll get. After being years of consultation with patients who reported a relationship of dependence and distress with cravings, I concluded this. Real food readjusts you at the hormonal and physiological level in such a way that you will control your appetite much better. However, this requires time and habit.

However, if we get that hunger for something sweet, that craving, we can always make good choices to replace that insane processed food. Here we are not talking about strategies to lose weight. However, when eating real food, we will be consuming foods with lower energy density and more satiating, which can favor our weight.

The thought that we are "on a diet" with strict, restrictive, monotonous rules and with unnecessary and incorrect prohibitions (e.g., "fattened" fruit at night, whole grains and dairy are prohibited because they are "inflammatory," not having avocado "a lot of fat," etc.) can generate even more cravings. That's why you should relax, stop the myths, and enjoy real food. I leave you a list of the real foods that give me the best results to fight cravings and snack something:

- **Dark chocolate:** It has to be more than 70% cocoa. Better without sweeteners. Normally with 2 ounces is enough. Taste it patiently.

- **Nuts:** A big handful of the ones you like the mos (not fried and unsalted)t. My favorites are raw cashews and pistachios. Don't take the package, select the fixed amount you're going to consume, and save them in place. We can also use seeds instead of nuts (e.g., pumpkin pipes).

- **Natural yogurt:** It can also be worth fresh, beaten cheese, or kefir. One recipe I love is mixing natural yogurt with nuts, dark chocolate, and fresh fruit. If the craving is for something salty, you can have a piece of fresh cheese.

- **Fresh fruit:** It is difficult if we are used to the sweet taste of the processed ones that we find the fruit's pleasant sweet taste. That's because our palate has been altered. However, little by little, with repetition of the habit, we will recover our real flavor, and we will be able to taste any fruit with a pleasantly sweet taste. I recommend baked apple cinnamon and homemade fruit ice cream (my favorite banana) for the sweetest.

- **Olives:** They told you to get fat, but they cheated on you. Two large handfuls of olives or a whole cup are a rich snack, with few calories and, most importantly: healthy monounsaturated fat intake, vitamins, phytochemicals, etc.).

- **Homemade popcorn:** This can be a good substitute for chips' cravings (no oil or salt). In this study, popcorn was more satiating than chips and provided fewer calories (and fewer insane ingredients such as refined oils). Here's a video recipe to make at home.

- **Coffee:** Did I already tell you that I love coffee? Well, it can even increase the amount of a satiety hormone called yY peptide. YY peptide has an appetite suppressant effect and can help us combat those cravings. We can opt for an aromatized infusion or a hot chocolate (hot water, cocoa powder without sugar) for the most nervous.

- **Cinnamon:** Cinnamon is a spice that can camouflage the sweet taste. I use it for numerous recipes with fruits, natural yogurt, and even coffee. It is also an antioxidant, improves blood glucose control, and many more health properties. I recommend a certain cinnamon type.

Important: Meal substitutes, "satiating" chocolate rice pancakes, protein bars, and other processed women's fitness laden with sweeteners will not solve anything, just a small patch that also contains insane ingredients.

Real Protein-Rich Foods

If we still have a lot of anxiety about eating, we can use the extra satiety contribution that protein-rich foods have. Protein increases blood coating hormones, such as cholecystokinin, LPG-1, and the YY mentioned above peptide. On the other hand, it decreases hunger hormones such as ghrelin. This study observed a group of overweight men who carried two low-calorie diets with different amounts of total protein per day. The group that wore a protein-rich diet (25% vs. 14% of calories) reduced cravings by 60% and desired sweets at dinner.

If our cravings appear mainly in the middle of the morning, breakfast should be the most protein-rich meal of the day. In a study in adolescents, a protein-rich breakfast significantly reduced cravings. An example could be scrambled eggs.

This meta-analysis of controlled trials supports real (unprocessed) dairy consumption as a good group of foods to improve satiety when on a diet and preserve muscle mass. For example, a satiating snack with good protein content would be natural yogurt with nuts. Some of the fat in dairy and nuts is not absorbed, so they are not as caloric as they are painted. Important: A serious mistake is to think that only animal protein is satiating when we know that plant protein, for example, of legumes, can have an even greater effect on satiety than beef and pork.

One of the main problems with ultra-processed cravings is that they are binge-generating. That is, you start eating out of control, and you can't stop. Psychologists who specialize in eating disorders recommend a technique called "conscious eating" or "Mindful eating." Conscious eating uses mindfulness techniques to detect and be aware of experiences, cravings, and physical cues when we're eating. This technique involves:

- Eat slowly and without distractions such as TV, mobile, computer, etc.

- Be aware of the physical signs of fullness that our bodies send us and stop eating when we receive them. Sharpen the senses by noticing colors, smells, sounds, textures, and tastes. Chew, taste, and think about food while we eat.

- Careful eating has been shown to reduce the amount of food during binging drastically and the frequency of binge eating itself. In this other study, after a 6-week group intervention in obese women, compulsive binge episodes decreased from 4 to 1.5 times per week.

- The severity of each episode is also reduced by 62%, so we're talking about a fairly effective intervention. If, in your case, you need professional psychology to help you with this tool, do not hesitate to go.

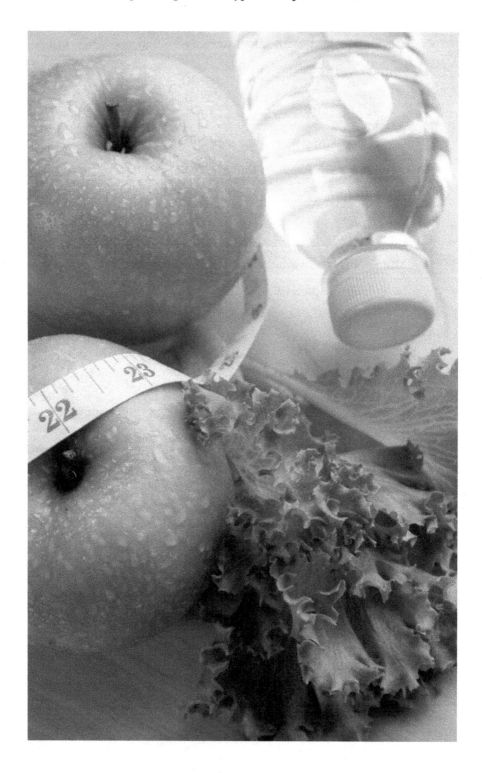

Conclusion

Eating disorders are one of the evils afflicting generations of young women and also of many men, but getting out of it is not impossible!

We need support, determination, and even a lot of willpower. In our opinion, it also takes an awareness that getting out of it could depend on us.

As we always say: you have to wait to "snap the chip" into the brain and understand that this kind of eating disorder does not resolve with a diet. It's a constant relationship with food.

It's often a struggle, as we like to say. But with an enemy that in itself is not a real enemy, if not a projection of our fears. Dig inside to solve problems on the "surface."

In conclusion, the stress response is a formidable capacity of our organism. It developed thousands of years ago to face challenges (hunting/defending) that today in our culture, we meet very difficult. It is calibrated for momentary efforts and defined over time, certainly not the normal state of activation. Therefore, it is necessary to learn how to manage stress and, above all, to turn off its reactions when they are useless. To combat mental and physical stress, we never forget that we are a mind-body unit: they influence each other incisively.

Practice conscious feeding. Conscious feeding is merely enjoying your food. It's paying full attention to what you do and savoring every bite. Take your time to eat, feel the textures, smell the food. All this will make you fully enjoy that you find real pleasure in eating again, and you will realize that you even feel satisfied with less food and start choosing healthier foods.

I hope this entry will help you re-establish the relationship with food and your own body. Tell me what you would like to accomplish to improve the relationship with food and whether you've ever eaten compulsively?

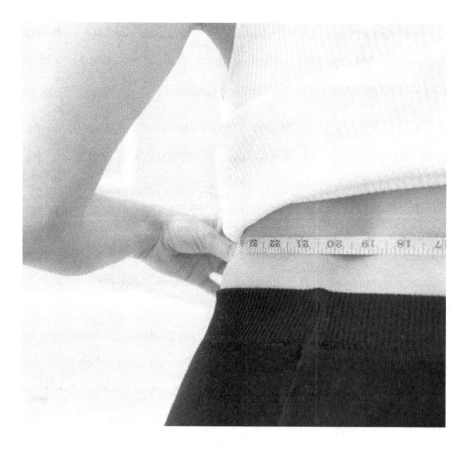

CPSIA information can be obtained
at www.ICGtesting.com
Printed in the USA
BVHW040918100621
609274BV00013B/3154